What you really need to know about

HORMONE REPLACEMENT THERAPY

Dr Robert Buckman

with Wendy Dear

Introduced by John Cleese

MARSHALL PUBLISHING • LONDON

A Marshall Edition
Conceived by Marshall Editions
The Orangery
161 New Bond Street
London W1Y 9PA

Edited and designed by Phoebus Editions, 72-80 Leather Lane, London EC1N 7TR

First published in the UK in 1999 by
Marshall Publishing Ltd
Copyright © 1999 Marshall Editions Developments Ltd

ISBN: 1-84028-249-5

Originated in Italy by Articolor
Printed in and bound in Italy by New Interlitho

Project Editor Alison Murdoch
Additional Editing Jill Cropper
Indexer Stephen Fall
Art Editor Louise Morley
Illustrator Coral Mula
Picture Research Carina Dvorak
Managing Editor Anne Yelland
Managing Art Editor Helen Spencer
Editorial Director Ellen Dupont
Art Director Dave Goodman
Editorial Coordinator Becca Clunes
Production Nikki Ingram, Anna Pauletti

The consultant for this book was Eva Kalmus MA, MRCGP, DGM, DFFP, Dip.Occ.Med, a
London GP who helps to run a community-based menopause clinic. She has three children
and is currently working in occupational medicine.

Contents

Foreword

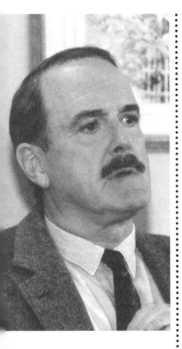

Most of you know me best as someone who makes people laugh.

But for 30 years I've also been involved with communicating information. And one particular area in which communication often breaks down is the doctor/patient relationship. We have all come across doctors who fail to communicate clearly, using complex medical terms when a simple explanation would do, and dismiss us with a "come back in a month if you still feel unwell". Fortunately I met Dr Robert Buckman.

Rob is one of North America's leading experts on cancer, but far more importantly he is a doctor who believes that hiding behind medical jargon is unhelpful and unprofessional. He wants his patients to understand what is wrong with them, and spends many hours with them—and their families and close friends—making sure they understand everything. Together we created a series of videos, with the jargon-free title *Videos for Patients*. Their success has prompted us to write books that explore medical conditions in the same clear, simple terms.

This book is one of a series that will tell you all you need to know about your condition. It assumes nothing. If you have a helpful, honest, communicative doctor, you will find here the extra information that he or she simply may not have time to tell you. If you are less fortunate, this book will help to give you a much clearer picture of your situation.

More importantly—and this was a major factor in the success of the videos—you can access the information here again and again. Turn back, read over, until you really know what your doctor's diagnosis means. In addition, because in the middle of a consultation you may not think of everything you would like to ask your doctor, you can also use the book to help you formulate the questions you would like to discuss with him or her.

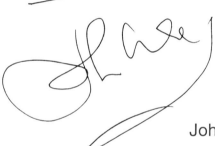

John Cleese

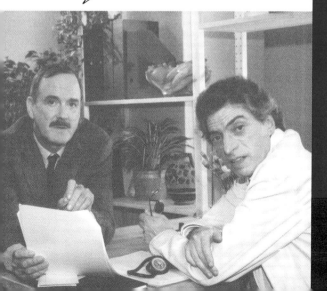

Introduction

Find out as much as you can about the subject so you can make an informed choice about HRT.

Don't be afraid to ask questions and seek help.

Hormone replacement therapy has a long history but for the last 20 years or so it has offered women the chance to make the change from one stage of life to the next much easier. The menopause is a fact of life for every woman born yet each one may have a different experience at this time. One purpose of HRT is to help a woman manage the change well.

The menopause marks the end of a woman's child-bearing years and the beginning of a new chapter in her life. A woman who reaches the age of 50 today may live for another 30 or more years during which time her status and activities may alter considerably. Another purpose of HRT is to help a woman to good health in her later years.

Information and support

During the reproductive years, whether a woman has children or not, her health concerns tend to relate to the way her hormones function. These give her body vital protection though she may not be fully aware of it until the menopause arrives and the symptoms of a lack of hormones are noticed. The prime female hormone, oestrogen, is fascinating. As more and more research is done its complicated, and highly important, role in the health of the body is revealed.

HRT is primarily a preventative health measure, used to protect the body against the disabling illnesses which can appear in later years. You will read more about each of them in the pages of this book.

So how do you decide about HRT? How do you balance the risks against the benefits? It must be an individual decision based on the best information you can get. The right doctors and nurses can help you decide how to make the choice by looking closely at your own situation. This book will arm you for such discussions. You will know more about what is happening to your body at this time and what may happen in the future if you have certain risk factors.

You will also have the information you need about the different types of HRT, how they work and what you can expect from them. With HRT no decision need ever be final. The choice can be made at any age. With the information provided by this book you become a partner in your own treatment.

A normal life

Remaining as well as you can be will be one of your prime concerns after the menopause, for this ensures your independence as you get older. Whether or not to use HRT is one of the decisions you will need to make about your health and quality of life in the years ahead. It may be as important as good nutrition and exercise.

This is a time of new beginnings. You may become a grandmother, may take up opportunities to travel, study or pursue other new challenges. The years after the menopause should be yours to enjoy, in health.

NATIONAL OSTEOPOROSIS SOCIETY

This charity has worked tirelessly over many years to make people more aware of one of the UK's most debilitating problems. It is a constant source of help for anyone needing information and advice.

Chapter

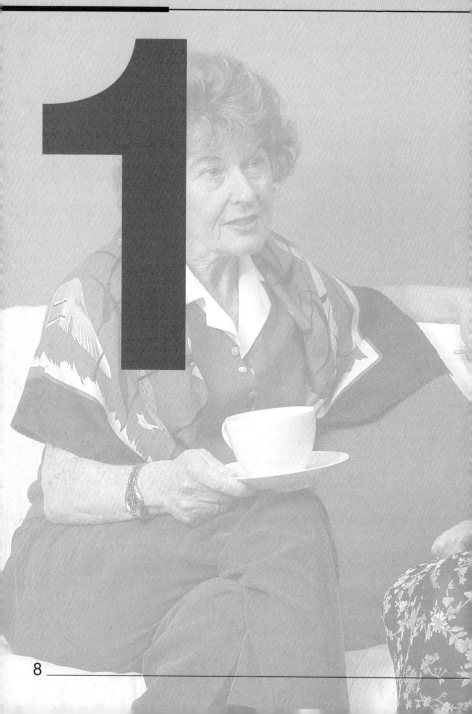

SYMPTOMS & CAUSES

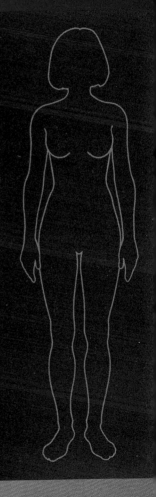

What is the menopause?

✓ Most women reach menopause a year either side of 51.

✓ The World Health Organization defines menopause as the date of the final period, diagnosed retrospectively one year later.

✓ In most women the whole process takes about four years.

✗ The timing of the menopause cannot be predicted—but some women will have experiences similar to their mother's.

The menopause occurs when a woman's ovaries produce no more eggs to be fertilized and the uterus stops its preparations for receiving them. It is one of her normal life processes and signals the end of the reproductive phase of her life that began at puberty.

What causes the menopause?

Towards the end of a woman's reproductive years, her body starts to slow production of the two hormones vital to natural reproduction—oestrogen and progesterone. As production of these hormones decreases, the ovaries gradually shrink until they are the grape-like size they were before puberty.

It is relatively rare for the menopause to happen suddenly. It is more likely to be a gradual process during which menstruation is irregular and eventually ceases. The time span in which this occurs is called the climacteric (commonly called the change of life), and the perimenopause is the time closest to a woman's last menstrual period.

For over 95 percent of women the average age is 51. Women who smoke may begin the transition at an earlier age and their climacteric may be shorter.

What causes early menopause?

Very early menopause, before the age of 40, may occur as a result of medical or surgical treatment. This may be after having both ovaries removed, after a hysterectomy in which one or both ovaries are left in place and the uterus is removed, or after chemotherapy or radiotherapy has been used to treat a malignant disease.

Very early menopause can sometimes also happen spontaneously, and the cause is not always discovered.

HORMONES AND MENSTRUATION

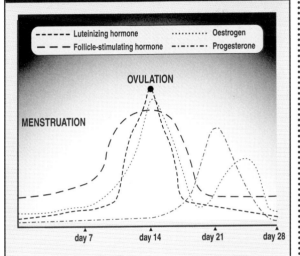

- - - - - Luteinizing hormone
- - - Follicle-stimulating hormone
.... Oestrogen
-- - -- - Progesterone

OVULATION

MENSTRUATION

day 7   day 14   day 21   day 28

Between puberty and the menopause the monthly cycle is affected by four related hormones, whose levels all fluctuate during the cycle. The function of two of these—the gonadotrophins—is to stimulate the production of two other hormones, oestrogen and progesterone.

HORMONE INTERACTION

In the first two weeks of a menstrual cycle, follicle stimulating hormone (FSH) helps an egg cell in the ovary to mature. When the egg is ready to break out of its follicle, the amount of FSH reduces as luteinizing hormone (LH) takes over to complete the process called ovulation—the point at which the egg is released.

By the time a woman reaches the menopause, few eggs remain, and the hormone levels tend to fluctuate more wildly, which causes periods to be irregular.

YOU REALLY NEED TO KNOW

< Even after many months without periods a woman is not necessarily "baby proof" so you should continue using birth control until you are sure you are past the menopause.

< Generally you are considered to be "safe" two years after your final period if under 50, or one year after your final period if over 50.

< Menopausal or "change-of-life" babies tend to be born to mothers who neither know they are pregnant or ever thought they could be again.

What is the menopause?

The effects of menopause

Menopause is not an illness, but an important stage of a woman's life. However, the hormonal changes that take place at this time can have long-term effects on health in later life. Oestrogen receptors have been found on nearly all tissues within the body and changing levels of oestrogen have widespread effects. Many of these effects have yet to be fully studied but information is available on the bones and the circulation (see p. 42). Knowing what could happen to these vital parts will help you understand why hormone replacement therapy is considered a great advance in preventative medicine.

How are bones affected?

Osteoporosis is a condition in which the bones become porous and liable to fracture. Bones—like the rest of our bodies—consist of living tissue that breaks down and is constantly renewed. The two reproductive hormones—

THE EFFECTS OF OSTEOPOROSIS

There are half a million tiny sites in the body where bone is constantly being lost and remade. When age-related loss of bone occurs, bones can become weak and brittle. This loss of bone mass increases the risk of fracture, especially in the bones of the hips, wrist and spine.

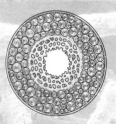

A healthy bone (above) has a strong outer layer of compact bone and plenty of soft, spongy bone rich in blood vessels in the centre.

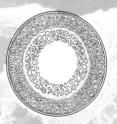

In an osteoporotic bone (above), the layer of compact bone becomes thinner and weaker and the spongy bone more porous.

oestrogen and progesterone—are essential to this process of renewal. Other hormones—calcitonin and parathormone—also have their role to play.

From the menopause onwards, women lose bone density rapidly and there may be no symptoms until they suffer a fracture after a trivial injury. Progressive spine fractures lead to severe deformity and pain, while hip fracture can be disabling and lead to loss of independence.

What gives bones their strength?

The strength of your bones is established in young adulthood through a combination of factors. These include a healthy lifestyle, a diet made up of a wide variety of foods and rich in calcium, daily exposure to sunlight (from which you obtain vitamin D) and regular weight-bearing exercise. All types of weight-bearing exercise, including brisk walking, have repetitive movements that place a strain on the skeleton and this in turn stimulates the bone-making process. The muscles also need to be strong to give the bones stability and help your balance, particularly in later life to prevent falls.

What can affect bones' strength?

Before the menopause several things can adversely influence a woman's bone mass (the bones' density and strength). The first is irregular, infrequent or complete lack of periods (amenorrhoea), all of which disturb the egg-releasing cycle (ovulation) and reduce the availability of oestrogen and progesterone needed for building bone. Period problems may be part of various illnesses, such as polycystic ovary syndrome and premature ovarian failure. Some treatments, for example those for endometriosis, may cause amenorrhoea.

**YOU REALLY
NEED TO KNOW**

◆ The body's bone structure is constantly changing and a person in the best of health should get a "new" skeleton every eight years.

◆ One in three women in the UK aged over 50 will have a bone fracture as a result of osteoporosis.

◆ The rate of bone loss is fastest in the first year after a woman's last period.

The effects of menopause

The effects of menopause

Can I minimize the risks?

If you are advised to have treatment that involves inducing amenorrhoea you should ask the specialist to explain for how long the periods will be stopped, the risks involved, in the short or long term, and what avoiding action can be taken to minimize the risks.

What else affects bone mass?

The eating disorders anorexia nervosa and, to a lesser extent, bulimia can also cause periods to stop. Over-enthusiastic aerobic exercising and athletics are another cause of amenorrhoea, and this type of oestrogen deficiency causes the bones to weaken prematurely. If a woman undertakes intensive physical workouts while not eating foods that contain calcium, such as milk, cheese, yogurt, sardines and broccoli, the mineral content of her bones can be badly affected.

Smoking and drinking alcohol to excess are also known to damage bone-building cells and to bring on the menopause about two years earlier than the average age of 51.

When are bones at their strongest?

Bones reach their peak mass between the ages of 20 and 30, the result of bone-making during childhood and adolescence. The level of your own bone mass will depend on several factors: the efficiency of the hormones involved, your state of health, your genes and your lifestyle. Failure to reach the optimal peak bone mass is a major factor in osteoporosis. From about 35 the bones are subject to persistent mineral loss, a situation made worse by the lack of oestrogen at the menopause and after.

Are there any warning signs?

Unfortunately the gradual change in the bones tends not to be noticed until a fracture occurs. A short, thin post-menopausal Caucasian or Asian woman who has lost height, particularly between the waist and the shoulders, or is developing a hump back, has the classic signs of the disease. Osteoporosis is less common in African and Caribbean women.

There are two types of osteoporosis, one of which appears at an earlier age than the other, but both are treated in the same way (see p. 31).

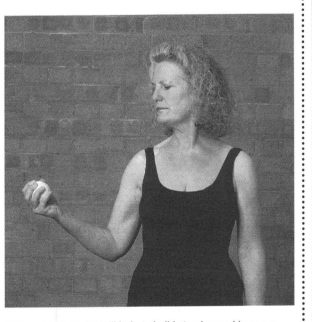

All forms of exercise will help to build stamina and improve balance but weight-bearing types, such as walking and the various types of racquet sports, are most beneficial for bones. Squeezing a tennis ball for several minutes a day is a simple but useful exercise to do at home, to improve both your muscle strength and grip.

YOU REALLY NEED TO KNOW

◇ Even if your mother or another close relative suffered from osteoporosis, your chances of developing the disease may depend on other risk factors or lifestyle.

◇ The bones that thin and get weaker fastest are the long ones in the arms and legs and the small ones in the spine (vertebrae), all of which are more susceptible to fracture.

◇ In older people, fractures are usually the result of a fall, often caused by a loss of balance, tripping over an object or confusion arising from taking prescribed drugs.

The effects of menopause

15

The effects of menopause

HRT is one of the most important tools available to help women at the menopause.

It may be essential to long-term health to make lifestyle changes well before the menopause.

It is rare for premenopausal women to fall prey to heart disease. Yet for women over 50, it is the single most common cause of death, just as it is for men. As life expectancy increases and people over the age of 50 make up a greater proportion of the population, medical attention is focusing more and more on this vulnerable area of the body.

Since the early days of hormone replacement therapy its long-term use—five to 10 years—has been promoted as providing protection against osteoporosis and cardiovascular disease (that is, disease of the heart, lungs and blood circulation). The evidence to back its role in protecting bone mineral density has come from many studies and while there are alternatives to reduce fractures, HRT remains the favoured treatment for the

OESTROGEN AND THE CARDIOVASCULAR SYSTEM

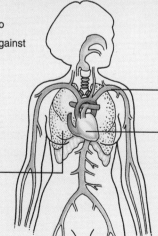

Until the menopause, the hormone oestrogen acts to protect a woman's body against the major diseases of the cardiovascular system: coronary heart disease and stroke.

Oestrogen prevents fatty plaques sticking to artery walls, so blood flow to the brain and the rest of the body is not restricted

Oestrogen keeps the muscular walls of blood vessels flexible enabling the heart to pump blood efficiently

The circulating blood carries oxygen from the lungs to all the cells of the body

prevention of osteoporosis. To be fully effective, however, it is thought life-long use may be necessary. With heart disease and stroke the picture is not yet as clear, and research continues.

Oestrogen and heart disease

It is known that during the reproductive years the oestrogen circulating in a woman's body prevents fatty plaques (atheromas) developing within the artery walls. When less oestrogen is produced, at the menopause, these plaques, which are partly formed by excess cholesterol, start to develop and narrow the arteries so the heart has to work harder to push the blood through. Heart disease—coronary artery disease—occurs when the powerful heart muscle is disabled by the restricted blood flow.

Lack of oestrogen is not the only factor involved in the development of atheromas. Your genes, general health and lifestyle habits also contribute.

Oestrogen and stroke

Stroke can happen at any age though it is most usually a condition of later years—that is, after the menopause. A stroke occurs either because something blocks the blood flow to the brain or because there is bleeding in the brain. Atherosclerosis—narrowing of the blood vessels in the brain or those in the neck leading to the brain—is the most common cause. The first sign of this may sometimes be "little strokes", transient ischaemic attacks (TIAs), which last a few minutes and may be felt as numbness or tingling down one side of the body. The risk factors for stroke or TIAs are the same before and after the menopause (see p. 42).

◆ Angina is the most common form of heart disease in menopausal women.

◆ Exercising and giving up smoking are among the best things a woman can do for herself at the menopause.

◆ As yet there is no clear-cut data about how effective HRT is in preventing either heart disease or stroke. But it is known that women using oestrogen have better blood circulation and can exercise for longer.

The effects of menopause

The role of glands

✓ A woman's sexual development is controlled by the glands in the endocrine system.

✓ Hormones circulating in the blood affect both well-being and your general state of health.

✓ The menopause is triggered by hormonal changes in the endocrine system.

We all have two sets of glands—the exocrine and the endocrine. The exocrine system is made up of a number of glands connected directly to various organs by ducts. It is responsible for the production of tears, saliva, mucus and sweat, as well as digestive juices from the pancreas and bile from the liver. In women it is involved in the production of milk (from the mammary glands), and in men the production of the fluid (from the prostate gland) that surrounds sperm in semen.

Glands and life-long health

The other system—the endocrine—is central to the way we grow, mature and have children. In women these glands produce the female reproductive hormones, often called chemical messengers, which circulate in the bloodstream. They have a strong effect on your general day-to-day well-being and life-long state of health.

The pituitary gland, about the size of a pea, works with the hypothalamus, part of the brain, to organize the endocrine system. In conjunction with the thyroid, they control metabolism—the rate at which you burn calories to provide the energy your body needs to keep every cell in a state of good health through repair and maintenance.

The thyroid gland, which is in the neck in front of the windpipe, regulates the body's heating system. It also controls the way calories are used and the level of cholesterol in the blood.

Very importantly, through its hormone calcitonin, it co-ordinates the building of bones, working with the calcium and phosphorus regulators and the hormone produced by the four tiny parathyroid glands (which are located behind the thyroid) to ensure the correct levels of both minerals in the blood for strong bones. (See also p. 12.)

A WOMAN'S ENDOCRINE SYSTEM

The different elements of the endocrine system have a profound effect on a woman's development.

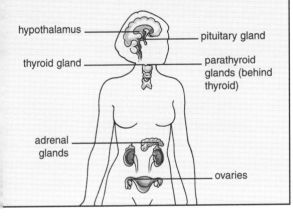

hypothalamus — pituitary gland

thyroid gland — parathyroid glands (behind thyroid)

adrenal glands

ovaries

How do hormones work?

The precise balancing act between the hormones is seen in the reproductive system, which, between puberty and the menopause, provides at least one egg a month to be fertilized. At the time when the pituitary gland sets puberty in motion, two new hormones are produced. The hypothalamus stimulates the pituitary gland to send out follicle stimulating hormone (FSH) to help an egg cell in the ovary to mature.

The follicle in which the egg grows releases oestrogen, to thicken the lining of the uterus, or endometrium, and luteinizing hormone (LH), which bursts the follicle to release the egg into the Fallopian tube. A cellular structure then forms on the burst follicle, to produce progesterone, which prepares the uterus for the arrival of the fertilized egg.

1

YOU REALLY NEED TO KNOW

◆ The production and ripening of eggs decreases between the age of 35 and the menopause.

◆ With fewer follicles to work on, the pituitary causes less oestrogen to be released.

◆ Unpredictable fluctuations in the hormone levels in the blood can be accompanied by infrequent ovulation, irregular periods and other menopausal symptoms.

The role of glands

Effects of hormone loss

✓ With falling oestrogen levels, many parts of the body, including the skin, bones and bladder, show changes.

✓ One definition of menopause is "the loss of ability to release a fertilizable egg".

In its role in the menstrual cycle, the female hormone oestrogen keeps the walls of the vagina moist and in shape, ensuring that the skin in the area is thick and well lubricated. From puberty onwards, oestrogen gives a woman's body its curves, helps with the distribution of fat on the thighs and upper arms and gives structure to the breasts. It also directly affects the walls of the arteries, preventing fatty plaques from forming and thus reducing the risk of coronary heart disease.

Does all the oestrogen disappear?

The production of oestrogen slows but does not stop completely at menopause. The amount that is produced depends on the amount of fat stored in your body. After the menopause most of the body's oestrogen comes from the fat cells, so a layer of fat is both protective and productive when the ovaries have ceased to function.

The quantity of oestrogen produced is much less than during the reproductive years, and oestrogen from fat cells is not as potent as ovarian oestrogen, which was stimulated by the pituitary gland. The adrenal glands (on the kidneys) also produce some oestrogen.

What happens to the progesterone?

If, after the menopause, your body is not producing enough progesterone (which is needed for proper thyroid function, including bone-making and protecting the lining of the uterus), you may experience the effects of having too much oestrogen. An imbalance between these hormones may cause what seem to be pre-menstrual syndrome (PMS) symptoms. It can also cause sudden weight gain or bloating, similar to that which you may have experienced during your menstrual cycle.

Fluid retention in the hands and around the stomach is not uncommon.

One school of thought considers that this imbalance of oestrogen and progesterone occurs as a result of the action of xeno-oestrogens (oestrogen-like substances absorbed through food which mimic the hormone). Phytoestrogens are plant hormones which also mimic oestrogen (see p. 22). Naturopaths say that a diet that includes plenty of these can block the xeno-oestrogens.

(see p. 22)

HOW THE BODY IS AFFECTED

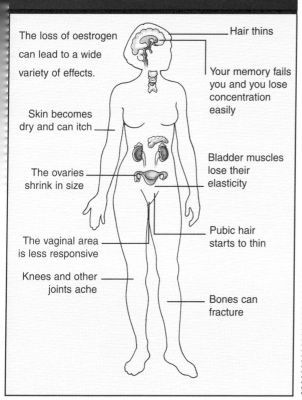

The loss of oestrogen can lead to a wide variety of effects.

Skin becomes dry and can itch

The ovaries shrink in size

The vaginal area is less responsive

Knees and other joints ache

Hair thins

Your memory fails you and you lose concentration easily

Bladder muscles lose their elasticity

Pubic hair starts to thin

Bones can fracture

Effects of hormone loss

Symptoms of hormone loss

✓ Without oestrogen, some body tissues, including those of the vagina, lose elasticity and shrink.

✓ Physiological changes after the menopause can make sex less pleasurable.

Lack of hormones can cause various symptoms, although some women do not experience any of them.

Physical symptoms

Dry, itchy skin is a common complaint. You may feel as if your skin is "crawling" or it may become sweaty and hot. Some women find they react differently to being in the sun and get heat rash or hives. Some find the deodorant they've used for years suddenly stops being effective.

You may experience problems with your teeth, such as bleeding gums, loose teeth or abscesses, and eyes may be dry and itchy. Your vagina may not lubricate naturally and be unresponsive, so that intercourse is painful. Even the thought of sex may worry you. You may have frequent urinary problems, such as cystitis, with

HORMONES AND YOUR DIET

Phytoestrogens are substances that are similar in their chemical make-up to natural oestrogen. Two of them—known as lignans and isoflavones—are found in many plant foods including linseeds, whole cereals and bran, vegetables, fruits, soybeans, chickpeas and other legumes.

These foods feature heavily in the Japanese diet and interest in them was aroused after studies conducted in Japan showed that menopausal women have a low incidence of adverse physical symptoms. Japanese women also suffer less coronary heart disease and cancer of the breast, colon and endometrium (lining of the uterus) than women in Western countries, although this alters when they go to live in the West and abandon their traditional diet. This low incidence of menopausal symptoms and cancers may, of course, be due to other aspects of Japanese lifestyle or genetics, and more research is being undertaken, but there is evidence that a balanced diet, rich in phytoestrogens, can be beneficial to women at the time of the menopause.

burning and itching, and you may experience "leaking" of urine when you laugh, sneeze or run (this mostly affects mothers whose babies were delivered vaginally). Your internal temperature gauge may seem to go haywire so that you feel very hot one minute and cold and clammy the next. Night sweats are common.

Hair can become thin, lank or oily, and the scalp itchy or bumpy. Your facial hair, which has been almost invisible until now, may become apparent around the mouth or along the jawbone. Odd, longer hairs can suddenly sprout from pores on the chin.

You may find yourself putting on weight, around the waist as well as on the hips, thighs and shoulders, and you may feel bloated and retain fluid, particularly in the week before you have or would have had your period. You may also feel unusual aches in your joints.

Emotional symptoms

You may find yourself more irritable than usual, or anxious about things that would not normally bother you. You may have difficulty making decisions and have feelings of unworthiness.

Your sleep pattern may go awry; you may suffer from insomnia or find yourself waking in the early hours filled with anxiety. You may feel depressed for no obvious reason and have difficulty getting your feelings back to normal or you may find it hard to concentrate.

Your memory may let you down and you may have to struggle to recall a person's name or a particular word or what you had gone upstairs to collect. You may suffer from unusual lack of confidence and mood swings, and you may feel unexpectedly tearful, yet your eyes may be dry and itchy at the same time.

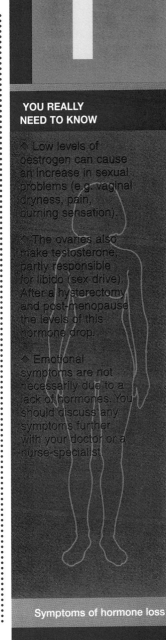

YOU REALLY NEED TO KNOW

◆ Low levels of oestrogen can cause an increase in sexual problems (e.g. vaginal dryness, pain, burning sensation).

◆ The ovaries also make testosterone, partly responsible for libido (sex drive). After a hysterectomy and post-menopause the levels of this hormone drop.

◆ Emotional symptoms are not necessarily due to a lack of hormones. You should discuss any symptoms further with your doctor or a nurse-specialist.

Symptoms of hormone loss

Symptoms of hormone loss

✓ **Give up smoking:** menopausal symptoms may appear several years earlier in women who smoke.

✓ **Keep a diary of symptoms to help** you monitor the way your body is reacting at this time.

How will it affect me?

You may get some, many or none of the symptoms that indicate the end of fertility. The physical and psychological effects may be severe and long-lasting or irritating and short-lived. In many cultures, the end of menstruation may be welcomed, because it allows women to take part in religious gatherings and prayers (from which they are barred while bleeding).

The menopause often coincides with major events in your life, such as children leaving home or relationship problems, and you may attribute your feelings to these events rather than to the changes taking place in your

WHAT A HOT FLUSH REALLY FEELS LIKE

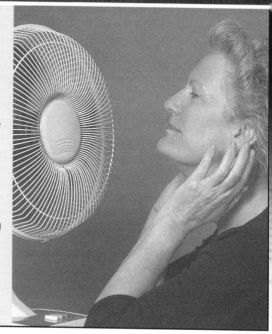

From the top of your scalp to the bottom of your feet you are suffused by heat then doused by a wave of sweat that feels surprisingly cold and makes your skin clammy. Several flushes may occur in a row, particularly at night, and you may become drenched in sweat. Daytime sweats, especially if they happen in company, can be embarrassing but the effects on you are not as noticeable as you think. Flushes are unpredictable and they can happen over several years.

body. Reassure yourself that you are healthy, that there is nothing unusual in what is happening to you and that the symptoms can be alleviated.

What if I am on the pill?

The oestrogens used in modern HRT are called "natural"—that is they are the same oestrogens (oestradiol, oestrone and oestriol) that the ovaries produce, but are artificially made. Women who take the combined oral contraceptive pill, which contains synthetic oestrogens (chemically different and stronger than natural oestrogens), may reach perimenopause or menopause without having any of the symptoms associated with constriction of the blood vessels (hot flushes, sweating) caused by changing hormone levels. This is because the amount of oestrogen and progestogen in the contraceptive pill is greater than that of HRT. In the past, the pill used not to be prescribed to women over 35. Now, however, the modern low-dose type is regarded as safe for healthy non-smoking women who are not overweight and have no other risk factors.

How can HRT help?

The purpose of hormone replacement therapy is to keep your hormone levels steady long term, to protect against osteoporosis, heart disease and stroke. Your body will function much as it did before the ovaries stopped producing oestrogen and progesterone, and because these hormones are being replaced you should not experience the range of symptoms listed on pages 22–23. There is a wide range of HRT available; some types cause a regular bleed, others do not. Only certain doses are considered bone protective.

YOU REALLY NEED TO KNOW

◆ If you are taking oral contraception and are around the age of 50, your doctor may take the opportunity to discuss the menopause and the possibility of using HRT.

◆ HRT does not make you fertile, so women who are definitely post-menopausal may experience the return of "periods" but are not at risk of becoming pregnant.

Symptoms of hormone loss

Chapter

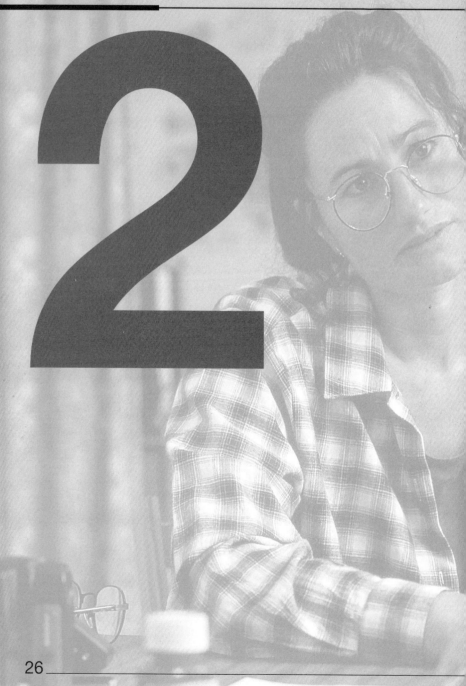

ASSESSMENT & DIAGNOSIS

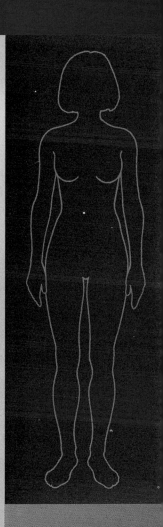

Tests a doctor **might do**

The ancient Greek physician Hippocrates, the "father" of medicine, was first to describe menopause, which he put at the age of 50.

For most women, the menopause is not an illness, but rather an aspect of their life-long health.

There are a number of tests your doctor may arrange for you to have to establish if you are menopausal and to check the state of your body.

Blood tests

If your doctor needs more information about your condition she may arrange for a sample of blood to be taken for analysis. A high level of follicle-stimulating hormone (FSH) in a woman under 40 could indicate premature ovarian failure; in a woman under 50 who has had a hysterectomy the FSH level might usefully reveal the arrival of the menopause. A woman over 45 who still has her uterus will not have her blood hormone levels routinely tested because they fluctuate wildly at the menopause and the results may not be of any help.

Blood tests may also be done to screen for blood clotting risks (if there is a family history of thrombosis) and to check your cholesterol level and liver and thyroid function along with a full blood count.

Cervical and breast screening

Women who are sexually active are advised to take up the national screening invitation to have a cervical smear test (either every three or every five years, depending on where you live). Breast screening is generally offered every three years, to women from 50 to 64. Women of 65 and over may request this procedure.

Ultrasound and pelvic examination

Ultrasound is a scanning method that uses sound waves to examine and take pictures of internal organs, such as the uterus and ovaries. If you have a history of period problems or fibroids, the doctor may arrange for an ultrasound to assess the condition of your uterus and its lining before further discussion about HRT. The doctor may also do a pelvic examination to estimate the size of the ovaries and the uterus. Without hormonal influence, these shrink and after the menopause they will be the same size as they were before puberty.

Bone densitometry measurement

This may be done if there is any risk of osteoporosis. It is most often carried out using a technique called dual energy X-ray absorptiometry (DEXA). If you have several risk factors for osteoporosis (see p. 40), your doctor may recommend that you attend a special unit at the hospital to have a bone density scan.

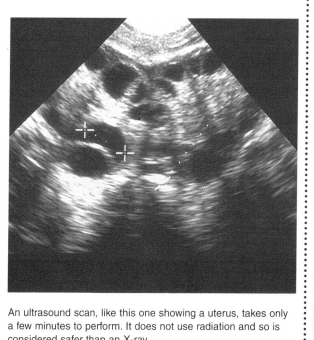

An ultrasound scan, like this one showing a uterus, takes only a few minutes to perform. It does not use radiation and so is considered safer than an X-ray.

YOU REALLY NEED TO KNOW

◆ Certain problems, which doctors describe as urogenital ageing, can badly affect your sex life at the time of the menopause.

◆ The thinning of the skin in the area may make the vagina so tense that sexual intercourse is either very painful or not possible at all.

◆ A form of oestrogen can be prescribed—as a cream or pessary or in the form of a silicone ring—to be used vaginally to relieve the symptoms of infections and vaginal discomfort.

Tests a doctor might do

Tests a doctor might do

The wrist is the most common site for a fracture in pre-menopausal women. This fracture, called a Colles fracture, generally occurs when the woman puts her hand out to break a fall.

Older women are more likely to fall on and fracture their hip, which is disabling and can lead to a loss of independence.

How is a DEXA scan done?

The scanner uses very little radiation and the test is simple and quick to carry out. You don't need to get undressed for it, though you should wear loose-fitting clothes and remove your belt if you are wearing one. You lie on a bed with your feet raised (so the lower part of your spine is flat on the bed) for a couple of minutes while the X-rays are taken and the measurements are recorded on a computer.

The computer printout, measuring the bone density of your lumbar or thoracic spine, femur (thigh-bone) or wrist against that of a healthy young adult woman, will

WHY A BONE DENSITY SCAN IS DONE

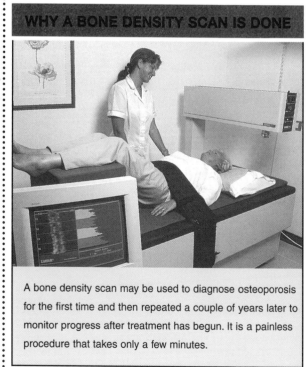

A bone density scan may be used to diagnose osteoporosis for the first time and then repeated a couple of years later to monitor progress after treatment has begun. It is a painless procedure that takes only a few minutes.

indicate whether the disease is present, if there's a risk of fracture in the future or, when combined with the fact of a previous fracture, show that osteoporosis is already established.

There are other tests that may be used more widely in the future to measure bone density. Broadband ultrasound attenuation (BUA), which concentrates on the mass of bone at the heel, is cheap to carry out and uses no radiation. Radiogrammetry (RA) can rapidly scan a bone, for example in the finger, and assess an individual's fracture risk.

What happens next?

The results of your test or tests will be sent to your doctor, who will explain them to you and tell you whether there is a need for any treatment. You may be prescribed HRT to protect against the development of osteoporosis, or other drug treatments if HRT is not suitable. If the tests show it is already established the options are hormonal therapy or non-hormonal treatment.

Once treatment has started, you may have a further bone density scan to assess whether the prescribed therapy is working as expected and whether your bone mass is stabilizing or increasing. Treatment must be continued for at least two years before improvements can be seen in bones.

At present there is no national bone screening programme for menopausal women, even though they may have a high risk of osteoporosis. Examining the bones in women with high risk factors is a reliable indicator. The tests may be offered on the NHS to those at particular risk or can be done privately.

YOU REALLY NEED TO KNOW

◆ A loss of bone density in women can be detected after six months without periods.

◆ New studies suggest that tooth loss may be an early sign of osteoporosis. After the menopause loss of teeth is common in osteoporosis sufferers.

Tests a doctor might do

Tests a doctor might do

Blood pressure measurement

Your blood pressure (BP) is measured as a matter of routine at the menopause, using a device called a sphygmomanometer. The nurse or doctor wraps a cuff around your arm, above the elbow. The cuff is in turn attached to a pressurized gauge. The nurse or doctor inflates the cuff to raise the pressure and stop the blood flowing. She then gradually releases the pressure while listening to your pulse through a stethoscope and watching the column of mercury on the gauge. Two measurements are recorded, when each of two characteristic sounds is heard through the stethoscope.

WHY BLOOD PRESSURE IS MEASURED

Blood pressure, in both men and women, tends to increase with age. While temporarily raised blood pressure is unlikely to be a problem, persistently high pressure increases the risk of stroke, heart attack and heart failure. As an increase in blood pressure may not have any symptoms and can easily go undetected, doctors usually measure the blood pressure of menopausal and post-menopausal women at least once a year.

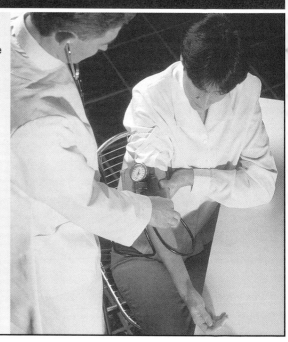

The first, higher, reading is the systolic pressure, when the heart muscle contracts, and the second, lower, reading is the diastolic pressure, when the heart muscle relaxes. These measurements are an indication of the forces on the artery walls as blood travels round the body. There is no such thing as "normal" pressure, but an average for adults is around 120/80.

What does high BP mean?

Pressure alters for various reasons. Running for a bus, driving a car, feeling stressed, smoking or drinking several cups of coffee can all affect it—as can anxiety at the prospect of having your blood pressure taken! It's best if you sit for five minutes and relax before the measurement is done.

As we age our arteries become less elastic, and blood pressure may be high for this reason alone, but a raised BP can also be an indication of heart or other problems. You may have raised blood pressure without any symptoms, and if your reading is above 160/90—borderline hypertension—your doctor may suggest ways of lowering it.

What can be done to lower BP?

There are a number of self-help measures you will be advised to take. If you are overweight you will be encouraged to change your eating habits to reduce your weight. You should also cut down salt intake and drink alcohol only in moderation (2-3 units maximum daily, see p. 75). Smokers will be advised to give up as the habit increases the risk of raised BP. A regular exercise programme can also help to lower blood pressure. If none of these work, you may be prescribed medication.

2

YOU REALLY NEED TO KNOW

◆ Hypertension means your blood pressure reading is above "normal". Hypotension means it is below "normal".

◆ Medication to reduce high blood pressure aims to control it without interfering with the effects of HRT.

◆ Low blood pressure is not usually considered a health issue and is rarely treated.

Tests a doctor might do

Chapter

3

CHOOSING &
USING

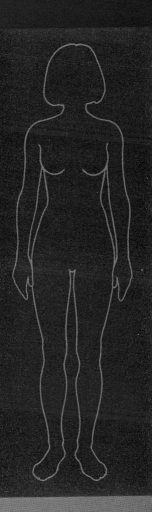

How do I find a clinic?

✓ Asking the right questions will reveal the importance of preventative measures to long-term health.

✓ Take your husband, partner or a friend with you if you think it will help you to understand the menopause and its potential problems more clearly.

✓ Note down the key points of your medical history and your symptoms before your appointment so you do not forget to mention anything that may be relevant.

You have various options. Your health centre may have a menopause or well-woman clinic, and you can always discuss the subject with the practice nurse, who should be able to recommend the best course of action for you. If your practice does not offer this service, the clinic time is inconvenient or you do not wish to go through your doctor, try your local family planning clinic, which may be financed by the local authority. Some run special menopause clinics where you can get information.

Special menopause clinics

You can pay to have a Menocheck with menopause specialists at a Marie Stopes Clinic (London, Leeds and Manchester). This involves checking your height and weight, urine, blood pressure, eyes, ears, nose and throat, heart and lungs, breasts, abdomen and pelvis, and reflexes. A cervical smear may be done and blood taken to check your hormone levels.

Private health insurance groups, such as PPP and BUPA, also offer checks, as does The Amarant Trust (an independent medical charity set up to promote greater understanding of the menopause and HRT and to support and extend research). The cost varies.

What should happen at a clinic?

Ideally you will see a doctor or nurse-specialist, who will have allotted at least 30 minutes for the consultation, which will take place in private. She will take your medical history, asking about previous pregnancies and contraception, if you have had a mammogram (breast X-ray) and when you had your last cervical smear.

She will also ask about the conditions you or members of your family have had, such as thrombosis, breast cancer, heart disease, fractures, thyroid, liver, bowel or gall bladder problems. You will be asked whether you smoke, if you drink alcohol and if so, how much per day, and about the type of exercise you do (if any).

You will be weighed, your height will be measured and your blood pressure taken. You will also have the opportunity to discuss any physical or emotional worries.

At this first visit you should ask as many questions as you want. It may be useful to write them down before you go. You will be given leaflets, and perhaps also a video.

THE FIRST VISIT

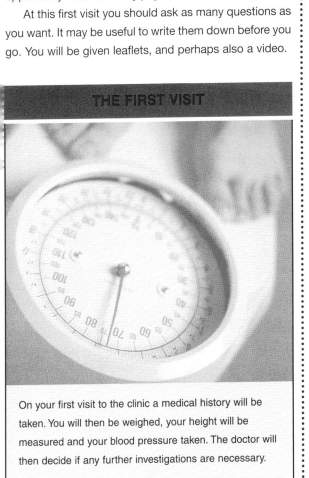

On your first visit to the clinic a medical history will be taken. You will then be weighed, your height will be measured and your blood pressure taken. The doctor will then decide if any further investigations are necessary.

YOU REALLY NEED TO KNOW

Questions you may want to ask your doctor include:

◆ How long will I have to wait for an appointment?

◆ How long do menopausal symptoms last?

◆ How will I know when I have passed the menopause?

◆ What are the potential risks of using HRT?

◆ What side effects should I expect?

◆ Will any side effects gradually decrease?

How do I find a clinic?

How do I find a clinic?

In the month before your appointment, record your symptoms, feelings and problems.

Don't be shy. Ask friends of your age for recommendations.

What happens next?

At this point it may be sensible for you to go away and read the leaflets or watch the video, then to make another appointment when you have had time to consider all the information. Or you may prefer to take the opportunity to talk to the doctor about the treatment that would be considered most appropriate for you. You may be asked further questions about the type of person you are and the kind of life you lead. This is important because it will help to establish the type of HRT that would suit you best.

WHAT MAKES AN IDEAL CLINIC?

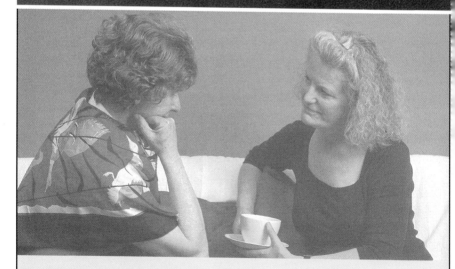

An ideal clinic has staff who have time for you and understand how you feel. They are willing and able to answer your questions, and offer up-to-date information freely. You are made to feel welcome and would be happy to come back after taking some time to consider all the facts.

Questions you may be asked at this point include: Are you good at remembering to take tablets? Do you object to taking medication? Which symptoms worry you most? Once the doctor has assessed your response to the questions she will tell you which type of HRT she thinks is most suitable for you.

If you decide you would like to start HRT, the doctor or nurse-specialist will talk you through the way it should be used and the signs you should watch for in the first few weeks. If you decide not to take up the option of HRT at this time you could discuss setting a date to review your decision in the future.

What if there are problems?

A good clinic will make sure you understand the purpose and importance of long-term, preventative treatment, and will encourage you to return at any time during the trial period (usually three months, but sometimes longer) if you are experiencing problems. If you are having difficulties with the prescribed therapy, it will be changed. This will continue until you have settled with a therapy you are comfortable with—tailoring your therapy to your needs and lifestyle is the best way to ensure your long-term acceptance of the treatment.

A good clinic welcomes both pre- and post-menopausal women and aims to help all women make an informed choice about the most suitable course of action for them. The staff will also recognize that the menopause can affect both you and your partner, and that you might want to bring your partner or a friend with you to discuss the options available to you. If your prescription must be written by your doctor, the clinic will explain the procedure.

YOU REALLY NEED TO KNOW

Questions you may want to ask your doctor include:

◆ What type of problems might I experience?

◆ Will I still have a period each month?

◆ Who should I go back to if the prescribed therapy doesn't suit me?

◆ How long should I stay on HRT?

How do I find a clinic?

Is HRT right for me?

Some types of gastro-intestinal surgery can prevent essential nutrients being absorbed, which can lead to bone problems.

Monitor your intake of milk and dairy products: women who do not get enough may lack calcium.

Women who are confined to bed through long-term illness are at greater risk of developing osteoporosis.

Your medical history

As you approach the menopause, or even once you have reached it, it can help to take the time to weigh up your possible risk of developing some of the conditions mentioned earlier. This will help you to make an informed decision, in conjunction with the professionals, as to whether HRT is right for you.

You know more about yourself and your family history than your doctor can ever know, but unless you have kept a detailed record of not only your own illnesses, but also those of close relatives, it may take some time to reveal it.

THE RISK FACTORS FOR OSTEOPOROS

Studies have shown that genetic, or inherited, factors, account for approximately 70 percent of the risk of a woman developing osteoporosis in later life, but other factors will influence the outcome.

GENERAL FACTORS

- ◆ Early onset of the menopause (before 45)
- ◆ A family history of the disease
- ◆ Prolonged absence of periods (six months or more) during the reproductive years (not including pregnancies)
- ◆ Long-term treatment with steroids (more than 7.5 mg/day for one year or more)
- ◆ Maternal history of hip fracture
- ◆ Asian or Caucasian background
- ◆ Long-term thyroid replacement (e.g. for thyroid cancer)

As these details could have a bearing on your long-term health, it is worth spending some time collating all the relevant information before attending a clinic.

Will I develop osteoporosis?

One of the most debilitating of illnesses in later life is osteoporosis (see pp. 12-15). If there were symptoms of it or it was diagnosed in your own mother, sister or father, HRT could be offered to you as a preventative therapy. Your own lifestyle will also have an effect. Check the risk factors listed in the box below.

The general and lifestyle indicators listed in this table also play a major part in determining whether or not a woman will develop the condition.

LIFESTYLE FACTORS
- Heavy smoking/drinking
- Lack of weight-bearing exercise
- Sedentary lifestyle
- Low intake of calcium
- Little exposure to daylight (vitamin D deficiency)
- Previous fracture (wrist, toe, ankle) after a minor injury
- Thyroid problems
- Digestive malfunction (i.e. chronic bowel disease, kidney or liver problems or after gastrointestinal surgery)
- Prolonged periods of immobility due to chronic disease

YOU REALLY NEED TO KNOW

Your doctor will find the answers to the following questions about your mother's health history useful in making a diagnosis about your risk of developing osteoporosis:

◆ Did your mother grow smaller in old age?

◆ Did she ever fracture a bone?

◆ Did she develop a hump back?

◆ Did she have an early menopause?

Is HRT right for me?

Is HRT right for me?

✓ Heart disease is the biggest cause of death in women over 45 in the UK.

✓ Using HRT reduces the risk of developing heart problems, but it is not yet clear by how much.

Your risks of heart disease

There have been a great number of studies, mostly in the US, on HRT and heart disease. But the results are not clear cut. In one, HRT users are 50 percent less likely to develop heart problems; in another it is 20 percent. The fact that over 300 risk factors have been identified puts the subject well beyond most people's understanding.

When you are considering whether HRT is right for you, there are two categories of common risks to look at: those you are born with, and those you can do something about. You can't change your genes and if you have a family history of heart disease you may have inherited the tendency. The risk of developing heart disease increases with age, and in women this risk accelerates after the menopause. Those who have had a very early menopause, before or just after 40, are especially vulnerable.

RISK FACTORS FOR HEART DISEASE

Your doctor can advise on reducing the risk of heart disease. Simple measures such as losing weight or stopping smoking can help, or you may need drug treatment for a medical condition such as high blood pressure (hypertension).

GENERAL FACTORS

◆ Family history of heart disease
◆ Age
◆ Premature menopause
◆ High blood pressure
◆ High cholesterol
◆ Being overweight
◆ Diabetes

LIFESTYLE FACTORS

◆ Smoker
◆ Sedentary occupation
◆ Little or no exercise
◆ Diet high in saturated fat
◆ Excess alcohol
◆ Stress

Next, look at your general health. The conditions which put you at risk of heart disease and stroke are: high blood pressure, high blood cholesterol, being overweight and diabetes. Finally, list the aspects of your lifestyle that may cause damage. Do you smoke, do little or no exercise, eat lots of fatty foods, drink too much alcohol? Are you often stressed, do you have a sedentary job?

Making changes

Talk to your doctor about how to reduce your known risks. Giving up smoking, cutting down your alcohol intake, adopting a low-fat, low-salt diet, losing weight and taking regular exercise will be the first recommendations.

Before the menopause, your artery walls have the protection of oestrogen, which also influences the level of blood fats (lipids, one of which is cholesterol). If you have an inherited cholesterol problem (called familial hypercholesterolemia), changing your diet to remove animal fats and eating more whole grains, vegetables and fruit may prevent an excess of the fat building up on the artery walls. Drug treatment can be prescribed if diet alone fails. One study showed that drug treatment used in conjunction with HRT had better results than either treatment used separately.

If you have diabetes mellitus—another high-risk factor for heart disease—and can get it under control with a high-fibre, low-fat, low-sugar diet or by taking tablets or insulin you can consider HRT. If you are overweight and can lose some of it all the better.

The role stress plays in heart illness is not completely understood. As the years around the menopause have their own physical and personal stress, finding ways to reduce its effect will always be in your best interests.

3

**YOU REALLY
NEED TO KNOW**

◆ Illnesses that affected your mother, father or near relatives may have an influence on your own health.

◆ There are only a very few medical problems that might preclude you from having HRT.

◆ If your condition can be treated and HRT would not be counter-productive, your doctor might prescribe it.

Is HRT right for me?

Is HRT right for me?

✓ The incidence of breast cancer increases as women age.

✓ All breast lumps should be checked by a doctor, but most are found to be non-cancerous.

Your risks of thrombosis

If you or a close family member have a history of thrombosis (venous thromboembolism or deep vein thrombosis/DVT) you will need to weigh up the risks against the benefits of using HRT. You can ask your doctor if a blood test, called a thrombophilia screen, would help to assess your risk. If you have no family history of thrombosis but if you are overweight or have extensive varicose veins, HRT may not be advised. DVT is relatively rare and the risk increases with age.

Your risks of breast problems

Many women have "lumpy" breasts during their reproductive years, others suffer tenderness or pain. If any of these seem worse around the menopause you should discuss the situation with your doctor. Lumps should always be checked out, although most turn out to be benign (not cancerous).

THE RISKS OF DEVELOPING BREAST CANCER

The risk of developing breast cancer in women taking long-term HRT is less than that reported from drinking two units of alcohol a day, smoking cigarettes or being obese after the menopause. Studies show that:

- after five years on HRT, there are 2 extra cancer cases per 1000 women
- after 10 years on HRT, there are 6 extra cancer cases per 1000 women
- after 15 years on HRT, there are 12 extra cancer cases per 1000 women

While this demonstrates an increased incidence, there is no evidence that there are more breast cancer deaths.

Also the small increase in risk reduces after stopping HRT.

Breast cancer is both age- and oestrogen-related. In particular, the less time a woman is exposed to her own reproductive hormones (from puberty to menopause), the lower her risk. For risk related to using HRT see the box below left.

If you have, or have had, ovarian or digestive problems, your doctor will take these into account, but they are much less likely to rule out the use of HRT.

Your risk of ovarian problems

Ovarian conditions often do not have any obvious symptoms and may not be discovered until a woman goes to her doctor with an apparent bowel or bladder problem. Cysts may be the cause.

If there is any hint of malignancy a hysterectomy with removal of the ovaries will usually be advised. At this difficult time a woman might like to seek the help of a menopause nurse-specialist who can counsel her. After a hysterectomy, she may be recommended to consider using HRT.

Ovarian cancer rarely has symptoms until the tumour is advanced. As with breast cancer, if it occurs pre-menopausally there is a chance it may be inherited. The risk increases post-menopausally.

Digestive illnesses

If you have had gastrointestinal surgery or any condition treated with steroids, your bones may have been affected, and this could influence the type of HRT offered. If a woman is genetically predisposed to colonic cancer her family doctor may arrange for her to be screened. There is encouraging research on the bowel-protective role of HRT.

YOU REALLY NEED TO KNOW

◆ Studies have revealed three cases of thrombosis per 10,000 users of HRT a year. The risk for non-users is one in 10,000.

◆ The risk appears to be greatest in the first year of oral therapy.

◆ Long-haul flying (more than four hours) increases the risk of DVT. HRT users might be advised to take half a tablet of aspirin just before the flight.

Is HRT right for me?

What about my weight?

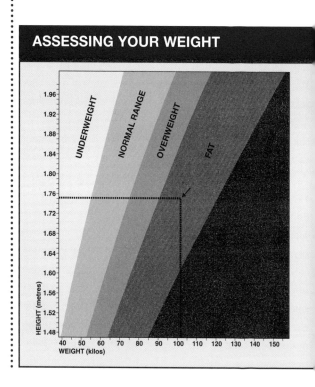

HRT prevents weight gain around the waist and abdomen after the menopause.

After the menopause the lean body mass decreases and the fat mass increases.

Your weight at the menopause is very important. Some "padding" on the body—on the hips, thighs and shoulders rather than around the waist (see p. 64)—protects the bones of the skeleton and is a storage place for vitamin D, without which calcium cannot be absorbed and used by the bones. Cells in this layer of fat also produce a weak form of oestrogen. However, this does not mean you should be overweight—you should try and keep your body weight as close to the ideal as possible.

How do I find my ideal weight?

Your doctor will weigh and measure you, then use tables to work out your body mass index (BMI) and the ideal

ASSESSING YOUR WEIGHT

weight range for your height. Some fat is needed to protect the bones from osteoporosis, so a woman with a light frame and no excess fat at and after the menopause, with a BMI below the normal range, may be at risk of developing the condition.

If you are at risk, a bone density scan may be done, and if the condition is diagnosed, treatment can be started. Treatment aims to reduce bone loss and the risk of fracture, with possible bone mass increase. HRT is effective in meeting all of these. If you have established osteoporosis, bone preservation is a priority. If you don't want HRT or it is contra-indicated in your particular case, ask your doctor about other options (see p. 68).

You can use the chart on the left to work out your ideal weight for your height, and to see whether you are within the normal range or if you are under- or overweight. The lines which meet in the area designated as "fat" apply to someone just under 1.76m tall who weighs 100 kg.

YOUR BODY MASS INDEX

Body mass index (BMI) is a ratio of your actual weight to your height. It is calculated by dividing your weight (in kilograms) by your height (in metres) squared. A BMI of between 20 and 25 is considered healthy. If it is below 20 it indicates that you are underweight and if it is above 27 that you are overweight. At both these extremes, your weight may be causing health problems.

YOU REALLY NEED TO KNOW

◆ The problems caused by being overweight can affect your independence as you get older.

◆ Wear and tear on vulnerable joints (such as hips, knees and ankles) is made worse by excess weight and can lead to osteoarthritis.

◆ After the age of 50, overweight people are at particular risk of diabetes, a disorder strongly linked to obesity.

What about my weight?

When should I start HRT?

If you start HRT at least a year after the menopause, period-free therapies should be chosen to protect the skeleton.

Young women who have menopausal symptoms after a hysterectomy should be counselled about HRT.

If you decide to use HRT, the only answer to the above question can be "when you are ready", and this should not be before you have been given all the information you need about hormone replacement therapy. The menopause is a normal event, a marker for the end of the reproductive years. However, a woman who reaches 50 today has every chance of living for another 30 or more years, and the quality of those years may be influenced by the changes that occurred in her body at or before the menopause. When you talk to a nurse-specialist and doctor about your health now and in the future, both with and without HRT, be as frank as you can, and discuss your feelings and any anxieties.

WHO SHOULD NOT USE HRT?

If you have any of the conditions listed in the left-hand column it may mean that you should not use HRT:

- breast cancer
- cancer of the endometrium (lining of the uterus)
- abnormal vaginal bleeding of unknown origin
- liver disease
- ovarian cancer
- deep-vein thrombosis
- pulmonary embolism
- otosclerosis
- pregnancy

If you have any of the conditions in the right-hand column, specialist advice may be needed:

- family history of thrombosis
- gall stones
- fibroids
- endometriosis (a condition in which fragments of the womb lining develop outside the uterus)
- osteoporosis (caused by the use of steroids)
- breast problems
- migraine
- epilepsy

You are much more likely to continue to benefit from the therapy if you have confidence in it, have made your own informed choice to use it and know that you have the back-up of people who are interested in your well-being. It also helps to know that if one type of HRT is not suitable for you, you can try a different type.

How long should I use HRT for?

You can continue the therapy for the rest of your life, provided you see a doctor for regular check-ups. When properly administered, HRT is free of major side effects and will continue to provide protection against osteoporosis and problems related to low oestrogen. If you use HRT after the age of 64, when screening of breasts and cervix is no longer offered on a regular basis, your doctor may arrange for you to be screened.

Will I need to change my therapy?

The range of HRT available is constantly expanding, and your needs may change over time. It may be that the type of therapy you were prescribed at, say, the perimenopause is not the best at a later age. Making at least annual visits to your doctor and nurse-specialist, who keep up to date with all the new formulations, is the best way of finding out if you need to change.

If you were prescribed HRT at the menopause and stopped using it after a short time, you may decide to start afresh later. Much will depend on whether there have been any major changes in your health during this time. See your doctor and nurse-specialist for advice on what is best for you. Whatever you do, don't just "give it a go" and then give up. Try it for three months and seek further medical advice if you are not happy.

YOU REALLY NEED TO KNOW

◆ Making the decision to start using HRT should be based on knowledge of your own health and what can affect it.

◆ If you have realistic expectations of HRT you are more likely to continue to use it and to reap the long-term benefits.

◆ A woman who has had a premature menopause as the result of treatment for an illness needs to know if she should consider HRT.

When should I start HRT?

Types of HRT

Various forms of hormone replacement therapy meet different needs. In a perimenopausal woman who has a uterus, two hormones are used so that the uterus is kept healthy by mimicking the hormone output of the reproductive years. The difference is that with HRT, the shedding of the womb lining as a monthly bleed generally occurs at a regular, predictable time. Or it may not occur at all if you are over 54.

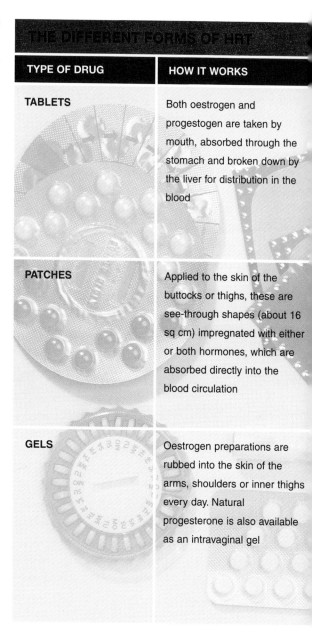

THE DIFFERENT FORMS OF HRT

TYPE OF DRUG	HOW IT WORKS
TABLETS	Both oestrogen and progestogen are taken by mouth, absorbed through the stomach and broken down by the liver for distribution in the blood
PATCHES	Applied to the skin of the buttocks or thighs, these are see-through shapes (about 16 sq cm) impregnated with either or both hormones, which are absorbed directly into the blood circulation
GELS	Oestrogen preparations are rubbed into the skin of the arms, shoulders or inner thighs every day. Natural progesterone is also available as an intravaginal gel

ADVANTAGES	DISADVANTAGES
• Simple to take	• May cause nausea • Hormone levels are not always constant • Require a good memory as lapses negate intended effect • Must not be taken by women with liver disease
• Hormones don't need to be metabolized by the liver • Various strengths are available • Hormone levels are generally constant	• Can be fiddly to apply • Need to be replaced at regular intervals • Apparent sign of therapy involvement • Do not always stick well on thin, dry skin • Allergic reaction
• Generally easy to use (five minutes drying time) • Amount used is self-adjustable to alleviate symptoms	• Not yet licensed for protection against osteoporosis • Can clash with some skin products • Women with a uterus must have progestogen as well

YOU REALLY NEED TO KNOW

The group you are in indicates which type of HRT will suit you:

◆ A Perimenopausal with a uterus
◆ B Menopausal, with a uterus
◆ C Have had a hysterectomy (ovaries removed)
◆ D Have had a hysterectomy (ovaries not removed)
◆ E Post-menopausal with a uterus
◆ F Post-menopausal without a uterus

◆ Groups A and B: oestrogen and progestogen
◆ Groups C, D and F: oestrogen-only therapy or combined therapy
◆ Group E: continuous/combined oestrogen/progestogen therapy but will not always be bleed-free

Types of HRT

Types of HRT

The oestrogens used in hormone replacement therapy—oestradiol, oestriol and conjugated equine oestrogens—are classed as natural (unlike the contraceptive pill in which synthetic hormones are used). The hormone progesterone is replaced by progestogen, a group of drugs similar to the natural hormone. If you have had a hysterectomy, you will probably receive only continuous oestrogen.

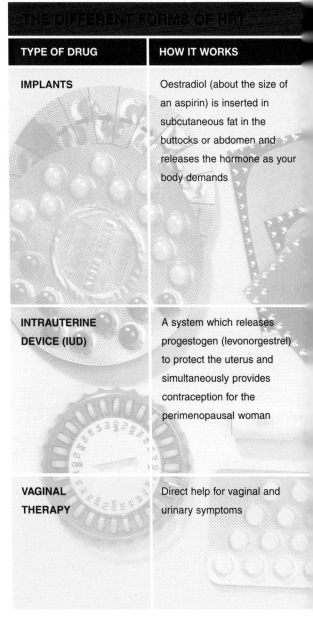

THE DIFFERENT FORMS OF HRT

TYPE OF DRUG	HOW IT WORKS
IMPLANTS	Oestradiol (about the size of an aspirin) is inserted in subcutaneous fat in the buttocks or abdomen and releases the hormone as your body demands
INTRAUTERINE DEVICE (IUD)	A system which releases progestogen (levonorgestrel) to protect the uterus and simultaneously provides contraception for the perimenopausal woman
VAGINAL THERAPY	Direct help for vaginal and urinary symptoms

ADVANTAGES

- Bypasses liver (therefore useful for women with chronic problems)
- Easily inserted (twice yearly, or less often)
- HRT effect may be increased by addition of testosterone to improve low sex drive

- Lasts up to five years
- Side effects rare
- Convenient
- May be used with an oestradiol implant (eliminating pill taking or patch changing)

- Wide range of methods (creams, tablets, pessaries, or silicone ring which is replaced every three months)

DISADVANTAGES

- Needs a locally injected anaesthetic and a small cut which leaves a tiny scar
- Oral progestogen must be taken for a set number of days
- Difficult to remove
- May require blood tests to check hormone levels (symptoms may return when hormone levels are high but falling)

- Has to be fitted by a doctor
- Awaits licence for HRT

- Not licensed for the prevention of osteoporosis
- Progestogen may also be needed in long-term treatment

YOU REALLY NEED TO KNOW

◆ An implant is categorized as minor surgical treatment and must be done by a medical practitioner. It is not always available in menopause or well woman clinics.

◆ Local applications of oestrogen are used to counter problems caused by ageing (recurring urinary tract infections, vaginitis and non-lubricating tissues which prevent or make sexual contact difficult or painful).

Types of HRT

HRT in tablet form

Hormone replacement therapy in tablet form is simple to take, but it is essential to follow the advice given with the packs, in particular when to take the tablet and what to do if you miss a day.

AVAILABLE RANGE OF TABLETS	
TYPE OF DRUG	**BRAND NAMES**
OESTROGENS	CLIMAVAL, PROGYNOVA ELLESTE, SOLO**, ZUMENON HARMOGEN** HORMONIN** PREMARIN**
PROGESTOGENS	MICRONOR-HRT, NORIDAY, UTOVLAN NEOGEST DUPHASTON PROVERA
ORAL OESTROGEN AND PROGESTOGEN (in right dose are licensed for the prevention of osteoporosis)	PREMPAK C NUVELLE TRISEQUENS CLIMAGEST ELLESTE DUET CYCLOPROGYNOVA PREMIQUE CYCLE FEMOSTON IMPROVERA
CONTINUOUS COMBINED (all are licensed for the prevention of osteoporosis)	PREMIQUE KLIOFEM, KLIOVANCE CLIMESSE ELLESTE DUET CONTI LIVIAL
QUARTERLY HRT	TRIDESTRA**

** Licensed for the prevention of osteoporosis

54

GENERIC NAMES

oestradiol valerate
oestradiol
piperazine oestrone sulphate
oestriol, oestrone, oestradiol (mixed)
conjugated oestrogens

norethisterone
norethisterone
norgestrel
dydrogesterone
medroxyprogesterone acetate

conjugated oestrogens, norgestrel
oestradiol valerate, levonorgestrel
oestradiol, norethisterone
oestradiol valerate, norethisterone
oestradiol, norethisterone acetate
oestradiol valerate, levonorgestrel
conjugated oestrogens, medroxyprogesterone acetate
oestradiol, dydrogesterone
piperazine oestrone sulphate, medroxyprogesterone

conjugated oestrogens, medroxyprogesterone acetate
oestradiol, norethisterone acetate
oestradiol valerate, norethisterone
oestradiol, norethisterone acetate
tibolone (see p. 71)

oestradiol valerate, medroxyprogesterone acetate, placebo

YOU REALLY NEED TO KNOW

◆ Oestrogen and progestogen tablets are packaged like the contraceptive pill so that you know if you have missed taking one.

◆ If progestogen is taken separately (with non-oral oestrogen), the first day of the month is a good starting date as it is easy to remember the set number of days to take it.

◆ A "tricyclical" regime" administers progestogen every three months and may be prescribed if a woman suffers from side effects related to progestogen. The aim is a withdrawal bleed every three months.

HRT in tablet form

HRT in patch form

Patches are small, clear adhesive squares that contain oestrogen (and sometimes progestogen), which is absorbed through the skin for a designated number of days. The hormones in patches are too low to act as a contraceptive.

PUTTING ON A PATCH

1. To apply the patch, tear the wrapper along one edge to reveal a small plastic square. Bend the square so one half can be pulled off the clear patch.

2. Without touching the sticky side, press the patch on to dry, hairless skin on the buttocks and pull off remaining half of the backing. Press on the patch for a short while to ensure it sticks.

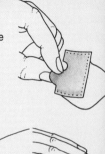

AVAILABLE RANGE OF PATCHES

TYPE	OESTROGEN PATCH WITH PROGESTOGEN TABLETS	OESTROGEN AND PROGESTOGEN COMBINED	CONTINUOUS COMBINED
BRAND/ GENERIC NAMES	ESTRAPAK 50** oestradiol, norethisterone acetate	ESTRACOMBI oestradiol, norethisterone acetate	EVOREL CON oestradiol, norethisterone acetate
	EVOREL-PAK oestradiol, norethisterone	EVOREL SEQUI oestradiol, norethisterone acetate	
	FEMAPAK oestradiol, dydrogesterone	NUVELLE TS oestradiol, levonorgestrel	

The patch should not be placed on the same area of skin twice in a row, nor should it be placed where it would be covered by elasticated fabric, such as on the waist or knicker-line, where friction might loosen it.

Your patch should not be affected by bathing, showering, swimming or exercising, but may leave a mark on your skin from the adhesive, in the same way that a plaster does.

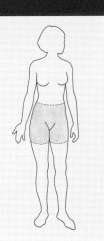

OESTROGEN PATCHES

(change twice a week)

ESTRADERM TTS & MX**
oestradiol

EVOREL
oestradiol

FEMATRIX
oestradiol

MENOREST
oestradiol

DERMESTRIL
oestradiol

ELLESTE SOLO MX
oestradiol

OESTROGEN PATCHES

(change once a week)

FEMSEVEN**
oestradiol

PROGYNOVA
oestradiol

** licensed for the prevention of osteoporosis

YOU REALLY NEED TO KNOW

◆ Patches are supplied in monthly packs marked with suggested change dates. The twice-a-week ones will say, for example, Mon/Thurs, Tues/Fri, and so on. You choose the days to start on. The once-a-week type will have the seven days displayed.

◆ If you are still having periods, the instructions will tell you on which day of your cycle to apply the patch.

◆ Mark the packet in some way to remind you to change the patch on the same day or days.

HRT in patch form

Other types of HRT

After a hysterectomy a woman can use continuous oestrogen therapy, as a tablet, gel, cream, patch, silicone ring or implant. A woman who still has her uterus must have progestogen to protect the womb lining. It is available as a tablet, gel, patch, intravaginal cream, pessary and a levonorgestrel coil, which is also a contraceptive.

LOCALLY APPLIED HRT

TYPE	BRAND/GENERIC NAMES	
SKIN GELS	OESTROGEL	oestradiol
	SANDRENA	oestradiol hemihydrate
	CRINONE 4% GEL	natural progesterone
VAGINAL PREPARATIONS	ESTRING	oestradiol
	ORTHO-GYNEST	oestriol
	OVESTIN	oestriol
	PREMARIN	conjugated oestrogens
	VAGIFEM	oestradiol
	CYCLOGEST SUPPOSITORIES	natural progesterone

LOCALLY APPLIED HRT

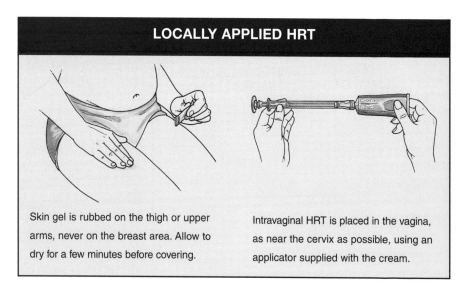

Skin gel is rubbed on the thigh or upper arms, never on the breast area. Allow to dry for a few minutes before covering.

Intravaginal HRT is placed in the vagina, as near the cervix as possible, using an applicator supplied with the cream.

3

HOW AN IMPLANT IS DONE

The life of an implant is generally six months. It is placed in fatty tissue of the body, usually in the buttocks but occasionally in the abdomen, in a minor surgical procedure taking about 10 minutes. The area is cleaned with spirit and you feel the sting when the local anaesthetic is injected. This takes effect rapidly.

HOW IS THE IMPLANT INSERTED?

A small incision is made and you feel pressure as a small tube is pushed about 2.5 cm into the skin through which a pellet of oestradiol is fed. Some testosterone may also be added to boost your sex drive (if this is one of the problems you have at the menopause). The tube is removed and a pad is placed over the area and held there for a short time to prevent bleeding. A plaster is put on, to be left in place for 48 hours until the wound heals itself naturally. A bruise remains for a short time and there will be a tiny scar from the incision.

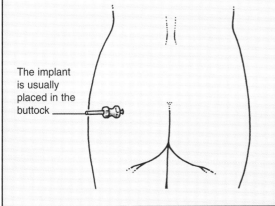

The implant is usually placed in the buttock

YOU REALLY NEED TO KNOW

◆ Period-free HRT, called "continuous combined HRT", was developed for women who still have a uterus and are post-menopausal. It provides therapy without "periods".

◆ In the first six months of the new treatment light spotting or bleeding may still occur.

◆ If the bleeding continues, there may be doubt about the date of your menopause. You may be advised to change to a sequential combined HRT (oestrogen followed by progestogen) for a while.

◆ You may be referred to a specialist if further investigation is thought advisable.

Other types of HRT

Chapter

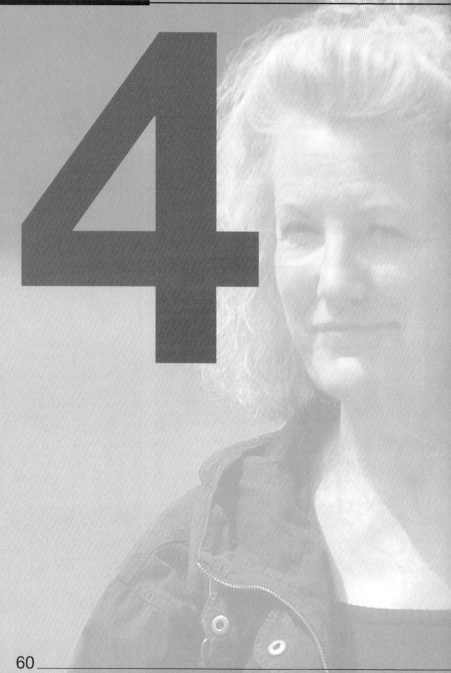

LIVING WITH HRT

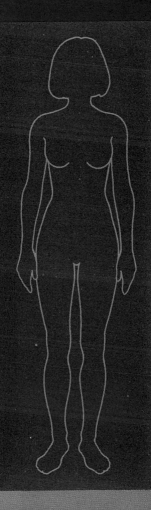

Your body and HRT

✓ While some symptoms of a lack of oestrogen appear at the menopause, others may not show until years later.

✓ Studies have shown HRT users have reduced incidence of age-related macular degeneration—the most common cause of blindness in older people.

Oestrogen and the heart

Before the menopause it is rare for a woman to have a high level of cholesterol in her blood (unless it is inherited, see p. 42). The female hormones circulating in the blood keep the levels of "good" cholesterol (HDL) up and "bad" cholesterol (LDL) down. Progesterone also controls the level of triglycerides (another type of fat), so the risk of atheromas forming is reduced.

Women who, before and at the menopause, have no sign of coronary heart disease may benefit from the oestrogen in HRT, possibly reducing their risk of developing it by up to a third. It is not so certain that secondary prevention (in women who have heart problems after the menopause) helps. If you are in this category, you can discuss your options with your doctor.

Oestrogen and the bladder

Urinary incontinence and urinary tract infection are both common at, and after, the menopause. These are uncomfortable, and often embarrassing, conditions which need medical attention.

Both result from lack of oestrogen (see p. 20), which causes the lining walls of the bladder and urethra (the tube through which urine passes out of the body) to become thinner, drier and vulnerable to infection. The tissues around the bladder neck also weaken, and this, combined with loss of muscle tone (a natural part of the ageing process), results in stress incontinence (leaking a little urine when you laugh, cough or run) or urge incontinence (the sudden feeling of needing to pass urine immediately). HRT may not improve incontinence in all cases; Kegel (pelvic floor) exercises may help (see p. 72) and surgery may be considered (see p. 73).

HRT and the cervix

The cells of the cervix change throughout a woman's life, under the influence of the reproductive hormones, but these changes slow at the menopause when the body's production of oestrogen and progesterone alters. However, smear tests are considered essential for women who have been sexually active. The earlier any change in cervical cells is detected, the more effective the treatment will be.

Cervical abnormalities are important at and after the menopause, when cancer is commonest. Hormones affect the cervix (making it more moist for instance) and the ease of taking a smear but not the abnormalities detected.

THE HEART, CERVIX AND BLADDER

Lack of female hormones has a crucial effect on some of a woman's vital organs.

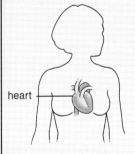

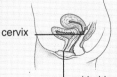

HEART
Without hormones to protect the artery walls, fatty deposits (atheromas) can build up

heart

CERVIX
The area around the cervix shrinks through loss of support tissue

cervix

BLADDER
You are more likely to leak urine when you laugh, cough or run

bladder opening

Your body and HRT

When a women is perimenopausal, fat on the hips and thighs is dependent on oestrogen.

At the menopause this fat is redistributed to the abdomen, which could explain why many women feel as if they are gaining weight at this time.

Gall bladder problems

Women are four times as likely as men to have gall bladder problems and they often appear in their forties. The gall bladder collects bile produced by the liver to help with the digestion of fats. Among other things, bile contains cholesterol, and if there is too much of it, it combines with mineral salts to form gall stones.

When gall stones are tiny and sludge-like they may cause belching, a bloated feeling and nausea after a meal. If they become large and pass into the bile duct leading from the gall bladder, they may become stuck. If this happens, severe pain, fever and vomiting may result.

Cholesterol and excess weight

Although the blood cholesterol levels before the menopause are kept in check by the female reproductive hormones (as is fat distribution on the body), it is thought

YOUR SHAPE AT THE MENOPAUSE

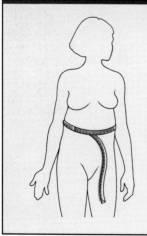

Some weight gain is common at the menopause. However, excess weight around the stomach and waist—commonly called an "apple shape"—means that you are at greater risk of heart disease and gall bladder problems. If your waist-to-hip ratio is above 0.8, it is worth trying to lose some weight. You can calculate your waist-to-hip ratio by measuring your waist at its narrowest point and your hips at their widest point. Divide your waist measurement by your hip measurement to get your waist-to-hip ratio.

that there is more cholesterol in the bile of overweight women. Putting on weight in your 40s could increase your risk of gall bladder problems at and after menopause and of later heart disease, particularly if the fat builds up around your abdomen rather than your hips and thighs. If a woman has gall stones or gall bladder problems, HRT is usually not advised until the problems have been treated.

A recent study of 13,000 adults aged between 29 and 59, conducted by the University of Glasgow, showed that anyone with a large waist size was four times more likely than average to develop late-onset diabetes and three times more likely to have heart disease. For women, the danger level is a waist over 89 cm (35 in).

Oestrogen and the mind

Like the breasts, blood vessels and other organs, the brain has oestrogen receptors and these may play a role in memory. The central nervous system, which is responsible for the senses of touch, sight, taste, smell and hearing, sends messages from the skin, eyes, mouth, nose and ears to the brain via nerve cells called neurons. There are gaps (called synapses) between the neurons, and chemical messengers (hormones) bridge the gaps to ensure the message gets through uninterrupted.

Lack of communication between neurons is a feature of memory loss and conditions such as dementia and Alzheimer's disease. Trials have shown that post-menopausal women who are using HRT don't suffer as much memory loss as those not taking extra oestrogen. And among women with Alzheimer's disease, the age of onset was later in those who had had some previous oestrogen therapy.

Your body and HRT

Side effects of HRT

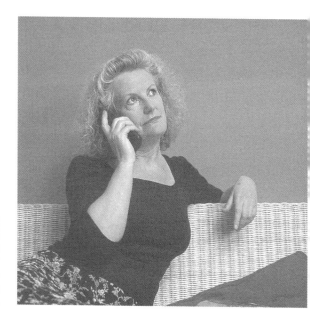

Before you begin HRT you should have had the chance to talk to the doctor or nurse-specialist about possible side effects.

Being aware of what to expect will prevent unnecessary anxiety and will encourage you to persevere with HRT, rather than stopping before you have given the therapy a chance.

When you first start HRT side effects are quite common. The reason is usually the sudden rise in oestrogen levels. For example, your breasts may feel tender, or you may have cramps in your legs, nausea or headaches. If symptoms persist, talk to your doctor.

PMS symptoms

If you still have your uterus you will be prescribed progestogen, which is given with oestrogen to protect the uterus lining. You may retain fluid and so feel bloated and you will have a period. This may not be the same as past bleeds, but you should be warned that it will happen.

You might find the side effects unacceptable, but don't just stop taking the progestogen—this can adversely affect the lining of the uterus. Go back to your doctor and discuss the situation.

If you are dissatisfied with your prescribed therapy, make an appointment with your doctor to discuss the problems so that a solution can be sought.

Bleeding

When you first start using continuous combined therapy, which is intended to protect the uterus while eliminating periods, withdrawal bleeding can be a problem (and may require the use of tampons, pads or panty liners). Bleeding can happen at unpredictable times and can be both irritating and inconvenient. This type of therapy is usually given for a three-month trial, so you should record the days of bleeding and report them at the follow-up appointment. If there is still bleeding after six months, action is required.

Problems with implants

Oestrogen implants are not as widely prescribed as other forms of HRT, but if this is the type you are using, you will have six months to note the effects. You should discuss them with your doctor, and if you are not happy, a higher or lower dose of oestradiol can be prescribed. The type of progestogen which must be taken for a set number of days each month can also be altered. Testosterone can be added if your libido has not improved. Menopausal symptoms are overcome almost immediately with an implant, and you know when hormone levels fall because the symptoms return.

The right therapy

If the chosen therapy is right for you, all your menopausal symptoms should disappear or be much less intense within days. After a few months of HRT you should have established a routine which feels natural and you should feel better. If this is not the case, go back to the doctor or nurse-specialist to discuss the reasons for this and to decide which of the other options may be more suitable.

YOU REALLY NEED TO KNOW

◆ The range of HRT is wide and new types appear often. When you have a follow-up appointment you may wish to ask about them.

◆ One of the newest types is tibolone, a synthetic combination of oral oestrogen, progestogen and testosterone (to improve libido). For post-menopausal women, it is taken continuously and does not stimulate the womb lining so there is no monthly bleed. It prevents loss of bone density.

◆ Irregular bleeding can occur when changing from another type of HRT.

Side effects of HRT

Treatment for osteoporosis

Hormone replacement therapy is licensed to provide long-term protection against osteoporosis, a crippling condition which gets worse with age. Healthy women in their 60s and 70s may be well past the menopause but can still use HRT or derivatives to protect their bones. If there are contraindications to HRT, other drugs and treatments (such as SERMs, see opposite) can be used.

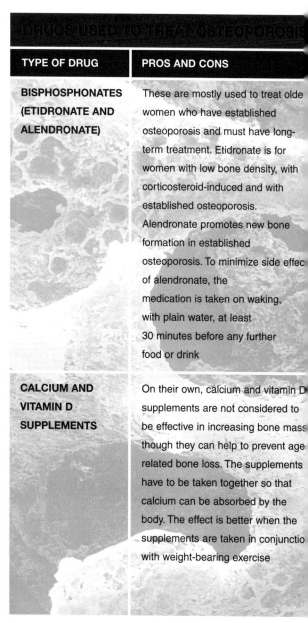

DRUGS USED TO TREAT OSTEOPOROSIS

TYPE OF DRUG	PROS AND CONS
BISPHOSPHONATES (ETIDRONATE AND ALENDRONATE)	These are mostly used to treat older women who have established osteoporosis and must have long-term treatment. Etidronate is for women with low bone density, with corticosteroid-induced and with established osteoporosis. Alendronate promotes new bone formation in established osteoporosis. To minimize side effects of alendronate, the medication is taken on waking, with plain water, at least 30 minutes before any further food or drink
CALCIUM AND VITAMIN D SUPPLEMENTS	On their own, calcium and vitamin D supplements are not considered to be effective in increasing bone mass though they can help to prevent age related bone loss. The supplements have to be taken together so that calcium can be absorbed by the body. The effect is better when the supplements are taken in conjunction with weight-bearing exercise

4

TYPE OF DRUG	PROS AND CONS
CALCITRIOL	Useful in treating corticosteroid-induced osteoporosis which occurs during long-term oral treatment for chronic illnesses such as asthma and arthritis. Rapid loss of bone density is a risk factor for people who take steroids for such illnesses
CALCITONIN	Given as an injection into the muscles. It is helpful in relieving pain, a feature of severe osteoporosis following fracture of the spine, as well as preventing further bone loss, though it is not as successful as HRT or the bisphosphonate alendronate at increasing bone density
SERMS (SELECTIVE ESTROGEN RECEPTOR MODULATORS)	For post-menopausal women with osteoporosis and women with low bone density. SERMs mimic the action of oestrogen on certain tissues of the body. They are not advised for women with current or a history of deep vein thrombosis and pulmonary embolism

**YOU REALLY
NEED TO KNOW**

◆ SERMs are for older women, whose bones indicate risk of osteoporosis, but who cannot, will not or should not use HRT.

◆ A SERM disables oestrogen receptors in the breast and uterus (which means it doesn't affect them) while working with those in bone.

◆ The SERM raloxifene (Evista) stops bone loss. Taken in tablet form, it has some side effects in the first few months, usually mild leg cramps and hot flushes. It does not treat symptoms of the menopause.

Treatment for osteoporosis

Regular checks

✗ For over 90 percent of women who develop breast cancer the cause is unknown.

✗ It is estimated that between 5 and 10 percent of cancers are hereditary, but it is not known, even with gene testing, whether those women at risk will develop the disease.

The breasts of younger women are "denser", that is they have more fibrous or glandular tissue, than those of older women. Between the ages of 30 and 40, the composition of the breasts changes and they develop more fatty tissue, which starts appearing amid the glandular. By the time of the menopause, most of the glandular tissue—part of the reproductive process—has gone. If a woman is using HRT, her breasts remain similar to those of a woman in her 40s as a result of the prescribed hormones.

In the UK, women's breasts are checked by mammography every three years from the age of 50. Before this age a woman who is premenopausal and considering HRT may have a mammogram arranged by her doctor if he or she thinks it necessary.

The purpose of these X-rays is to look for changes in the breast and to follow up anything unusual that may be seen. A woman going for screening will be asked if she is using HRT as this will help the radiologist, who reads the X-ray, to understand why the mammogram appears to be that of a younger woman.

The importance of early detection

Of the breast lumps found, only one in 10 will be cancerous and most will not spread from the original site. Early detection and prompt treatment have the greatest effect on this type of breast cancer. It is also thought that breast cancers found in HRT users are less aggressive and the outcome is better than in those who develop breast cancer when not on HRT. It is a fact that breast cancer is a common illness of post-menopausal women, but the greatest risk of death for them is heart disease. There is as yet no conclusive proof that HRT increases the risk of breast cancer.

Follow up

Once you are settled on your type of HRT, your doctor should encourage you to be checked regularly, at least once a year. Prescriptions are not repeated automatically and a doctor's appointment will be needed for renewal. Your weight and blood pressure will be monitored, you will be advised on breast examination and you will be asked about any side effects you might be experiencing.

You may also have a pelvic examination if there has been any unusual bleeding. You may be asked about your lifestyle (how much regular exercise you take, for example) and if you have not yet had the menopause the subject of contraception may be discussed and the date of your next smear checked.

HAVING A MAMMOGRAM

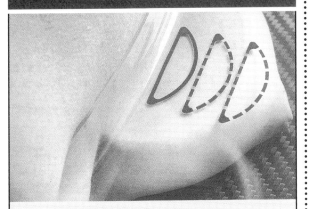

The X-rays used in a mammogram penetrate only a few centimetres into the breast, and so carry very little risk. Your breasts are compressed between two plates during the procedure (shown above), which can cause discomfort.

YOU REALLY NEED TO KNOW

◆ Studies around the world are showing that HRT offers long-term protection against osteoporosis.

◆ HRT protects against endometrial, ovarian and colonic cancers.

◆ HRT is thought to improve gum health and thus reduce tooth loss.

◆ HRT may improve balance and help to maintain memory.

Regular checks

Controlling incontinence

Don't suffer in silence: incontinence can be helped by exercises, drugs or surgery.

Incontinence gets worse at the menopause because oestrogen loss affects the muscles.

Some women suffer from urinary incontinence for many years without seeking help, because they are too embarrassed to discuss it. Yet it is exceedingly common, and doctors do understand the problem and the feelings it engenders.

There are two main types. Stress incontinence is the condition in which a small amount of urine leaks out when you are exercising or when you laugh, cough or sneeze. With the other type, urge incontinence, you just can't hold back the need to pass urine by concentrating on something else or crossing your legs. Both may be related to loss of oestrogen or can be the long-term result of

KEGEL EXERCISES TO TIGHTEN PELVIC FLOOR MUSCLES

These exercises improve the tone of the pelvic floor muscles and prevent "leaking". Do them as often as you can every day.

◆ Keep your legs slightly apart and close your back passage (anus) as if you were trying to avoid passing wind.

◆ At the same time, draw the front passage (vagina) inwards and upwards as if trying to stop passing urine.

◆ Count to five, saying to yourself "a thousand and one, a thousand and two..." up to five.

◆ Relax for a count of five, then repeat. The aim is to gradually hold the passages closed for 15 seconds.

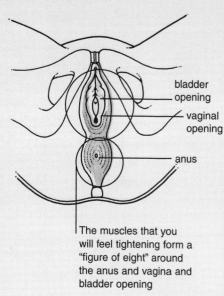

bladder opening

vaginal opening

anus

The muscles that you will feel tightening form a "figure of eight" around the anus and vagina and bladder opening

giving birth vaginally. Incontinence can affect not just your social life but your sex life as well. The return of oestrogen to the body through HRT may restore control in many women, but others may need more help to overcome the problem.

The doctor or nurse-specialist at a well woman clinic will explain the various methods that can be used. Ways of training the bladder may be suggested or medical intervention (e.g. drugs) may be advised. Doing pelvic floor exercises will be encouraged.

Is surgery necessary?

In some cases of incontinence you may be referred to a specialist incontinence clinic. In the past surgery has been considered the best option to tighten the neck of the bladder, but another, less invasive, treatment is now being used successfully. A collagen injection, done as a day-case procedure, stops the leakage of urine by padding out the tissue of the bladder neck. Pioneered by a urogynaecologist at a London hospital, the technique is helpful for women of any age, particularly those who would rather avoid major surgery.

Kegel (pelvic floor) exercises

You can keep the muscles in this part of the body toned by exercises. Pregnant women are advised to do them before and after the birth. The beauty of the exercises is that you can do them whenever and wherever you want (for example, queuing for a bus, sitting at your desk, vacuuming the floor) without anyone knowing. The improvement won't be instantaneous, but after eight weeks of doing them at least three to five times a day you will notice that your control is much better.

**YOU REALLY
NEED TO KNOW**

◆ Women have quite a short urinary tract and the opening is close to both the vagina and the anus so this area is prone to infection.

◆ The bladder holds about half a litre of urine, but if you get into the habit of emptying it before it is even half full, the muscle tone is affected for the worse.

◆ The pelvic floor is made up of muscles which form a "sling" that supports the bladder, rectum and uterus. In pregnancy the expanding uterus can put stress on the whole area.

Controlling incontinence

Lifestyle changes

One of the easiest ways to manage stress is by taking exercise.

A moderate intake of wine (up to a glass and a half a day) may give some protection against stroke and heart disease and may also protect against Alzheimer's and Parkinson's diseases.

Drink plain water throughout the day to counter your body's normal water loss.

HRT is not a substitute for healthy eating and exercise. While it is healthier at and after the menopause to have some body fat (see p. 46), being overweight isn't good for you. The World Health Organization and other health experts are agreed that by changing your eating habits you are likely to reduce your risk of developing heart disease, stroke, diabetes and some common cancers.

Vitamins and minerals

Vitamins and minerals make the body function at its optimal level. Nutritionists and dieticians say that you should get all you need from a balanced diet but you may not be eating a wide enough variety of foods or they may be altered by disease, processing or cooking. A diet or lifestyle restricted by illness or age, smoking or, rarely, taking medicinal drugs which deplete vitamin and mineral levels, can have an effect too (HRT is not in this category).

Should I take supplements?

This depends on your diet. As you get older the antioxidants (vitamins A, C, E and the mineral selenium) become more important to protect the cells of the body from damage. It is important to heed any warnings that may be given. Vitamin A should not be taken in excess and calcium can leave deposits in the kidneys. Bone-protecting supplements combine calcium with vitamin D, and calcium is formulated with glucosamine and chondroitin (both found naturally in the connective tissue of joints). Usually the body will excrete any calcium it doesn't need—as it will most excess vitamins and minerals—but if you are in any doubt you should ask your doctor or a nutritionist for advice. Supplements give the recommended daily allowance (RDA) on the label.

Move with the times

Inactivity will eventually lead to immobility. The best type of exercise will build strength and stamina, increase flexibility, and help your balance and concentration.

Improving bone density and muscle strength should be a priority at and after the menopause. The exercises, sports and activities which do this best are tennis, badminton, brisk walking, jogging, climbing stairs, step aerobics, trampolining and line dancing. Swimming and cycling, though good for overall fitness, are not weight-bearing. You should aim to breathe deeply and move well, both of which will lift your spirits as they increase your serotonin levels (a brain hormone that affects mood).

TAKE REGULAR EXERCISE

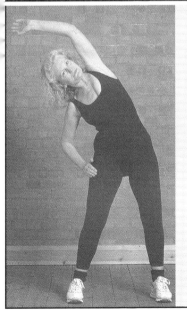

At the menopause and after, exercise should be a regular activity—30 minutes a day, or at least three times a week, is recommended to keep you physically fit. Some simple rules are: walk instead of drive, climb stairs instead of taking the lift, play a sport instead of watching it on TV.

YOU REALLY NEED TO KNOW

◆ Apart from improved diet and increased exercise, managing stress, stopping smoking and avoiding excess alcohol are considered the three most important contributions you can make to your own well-being.

◆ Drinking excess alcohol is linked to a variety of illnesses, including those of the stomach, liver, kidneys, breasts, bladder and bowel. "Safe" limits for a woman are 14-21 units a week. One unit equals a glass of wine or a single measure of spirits or half a pint of beer.

Lifestyle changes

Understanding the jargon

Many of the terms that you will meet when finding out more about HRT and the menopause may be unfamiliar to you. This page gives definitions of the words you are most likely to come across.

AMENORRHOEA—absence of periods

CERVIX—the neck of the womb (uterus)

CLIMACTERIC—the time during which menstruation is irregular and eventually ceases

CORTICOSTEROIDS—powerful steroid drugs which are used to reduce inflammation in the body

D&C—(dilatation and curettage) surgical procedure to scrape out or check the womb lining

DYSPAREUNIA—painful sex

ENDOMETRIOSIS—abnormal growth of the womb lining outside the womb

FIBROIDS—benign growth in the womb

FOLLICLE—sac for eggs in the ovary

FSH—follicle stimulating hormone produced by the pituitary to stimulate the ovary to produce eggs

GONADS—female (and male) sex glands

HYSTERECTOMY—surgical removal of the womb

ISOFLAVONES—weak oestrogen-like chemicals

LH—luteinizing hormone from the pituitary which stimulates the ovary to produce progesterone

MAMMOGRAPHY—procedure in which the breasts are X-rayed to screen for abnormal changes

MENARCHE—start of menstruation (periods)

MENORRHAGIA—heavy periods

OOPHORECTOMY—surgical removal of an ovary

OVARY—female sex gland

PERIMENOPAUSE—the time around the menopause

POLYP—growth, usually benign, in the womb lining or at the cervix

PROLAPSE—downward slippage (most commonly of the womb, neck of the bladder or lower bowel)

SPECULUM—instrument used to open the vagina for an internal examination or smear

URETHRA—tube that carries urine from the bladder out of the body

UTERUS—the womb, a muscular organ under the influence of the reproductive hormones

VAGINISMUS—involuntary paralysis of the vaginal area which prevents sex or internal examination

VULVA—describes the area around the vagina

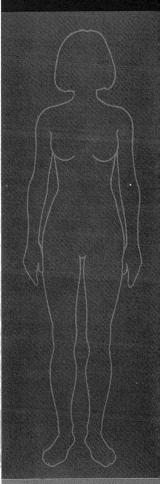

Understanding the jargon

Useful addresses

THE AMARANT CENTRE
Churchill Clinic
80 Lambeth Road
London SE1 7PW
Tel: 0207 401 3855
Treats women referred by a GP
or practice nurse. There is a scale
of fees.

THE AMARANT TRUST
First Floor
Sycamore House
5 Sycamore Street
London EC1Y 0SR
Tel: 0207 608 3222
An independent charity that
promotes greater understanding
of the menopause and HRT and
supports research.

**BUPA WELL WOMAN
SCREENING CLINIC**
Battle Bridge House
300 Gray's Inn Road
London WC1X 8DU
Tel: 0207 837 6484

MARIE STOPES INTERNATIONAL
Marie Stopes House
108 Whitfield Street
London W1P 6BE
Tel: 0207 388 2585
http://www.mariestopes.org.uk
Help in the field of reproductive
healthcare worldwide. No referral
needed to attend a menopause
clinic, but a fee is payable to
cover the consultation and
physical checks.

**THE NATIONAL OSTEOPOROSIS
SOCIETY**
PO Box 10
Radstock
Bath BA3 3YB
Tel: 01761 471771
Helpline: 01761 472721
A charity that aims to keep the
public and health professionals
informed about this bone disease.

PRIVATE PATIENTS PLAN (PPP)
Phillips House
Crescent Road
Tunbridge Wells
Kent TN1 2PL
Tel: 01892 512345

Index

Index

Acknowledgements
Photographs: Science Photo Library 12, 29, 30, 32, 42, 44, 68-69;
Tony Stone Images 26-7, 37, 70-71. All other photographs: George Taylor.
Weight assessment chart 46, Health Education Authority.

Thanks to Patricia Monahan and Wendy Dear for modelling for the photographs.
Thanks too to Jackie Parrington, Nurse Manager at the National Osteoporosis
Society for her invaluable help.